The Vibrant Vegan Air Fryer Cookbook

The Best and Healthy Vegan Air Fryer Recipes

Samantha Attanasio

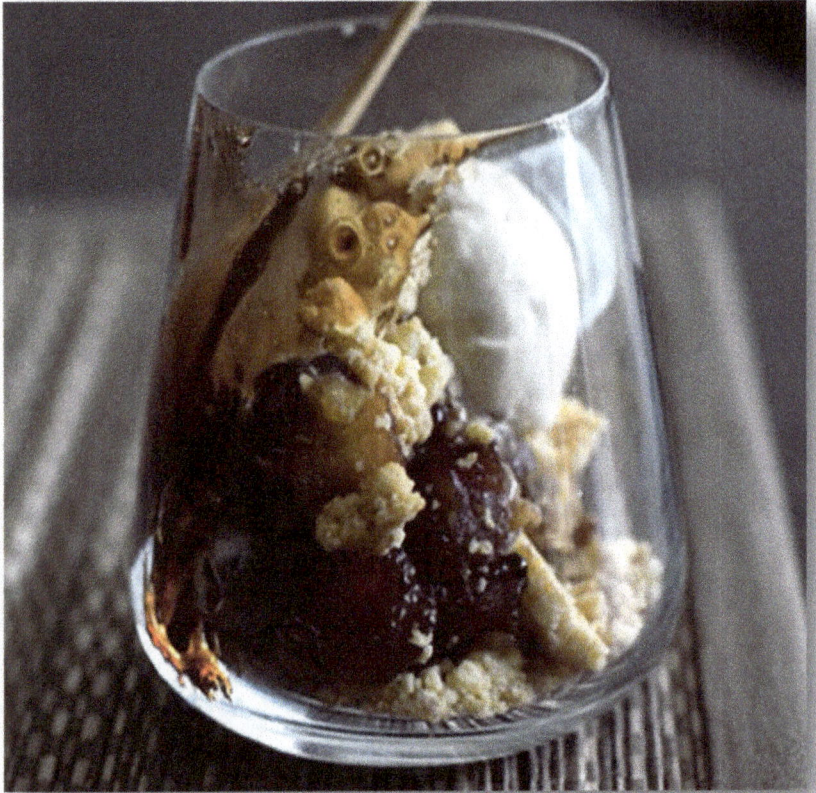

Table of Contents

Vegetable

Greek Potato Mix

Preparation time: 10 minutes

Cooking time: 20 minutes

Servings: 4

Ingredients:

- 1½ pounds potatoes, peeled and cubed
- Two tbsp. olive oil
- Salt and black pepper to taste
- One tbsp. hot paprika
- 2 ounces coconut cream

Directions:

Put potatoes in a bowl and add water to cover.

Leave them aside for 10 minutes.

Drain them and mix with half of the oil, salt, pepper and paprika and toss them.

Put potatoes in your air fryer's basket.

Cook at the set temperature 360 degrees F for 20 minutes.

In a bowl, mix coconut cream with salt, pepper and the rest of the oil and stir well.

Divide potatoes between plates.

Add coconut cream on top. Serve and enjoy!

Nutrition:

Energy (calories): 203 kcal

Protein: 4 g

Fat: 7.17 g

Carbohydrates: 32.22 g

Tasty Mushroom Cakes

Preparation time: 10 minutes
Cooking time: 2 Hours 8 Minutes
Servings: 8

Ingredients:

- Ounces mushrooms, chopped
- One small yellow onion, chopped
- Salt and black pepper to the taste
- ¼ tsp. nutmeg, ground
- Two tbsp. olive oil
- One tbsp. breadcrumbs
- 14 ounces of coconut milk

Direction:

Over medium-high heat, cook and heat half of the oil in a pan...

Add onion and mushrooms.

Stir and cook for 3 minutes.

Add the coconut milk, salt, nutmeg and pepper, and stir.

Take off heat and leave aside for 2 hours.

Mix the rest of the oil in a bowl, with breadcrumbs and stir well.

Take one tbsp. mushroom filling, roll in breadcrumbs and put them in your air fryer basket.

Repeat with the rest of the mushroom mix and cook cakes at 400 degrees F for 8 minutes.

Divide mushroom cakes between plates. Serve and enjoy!

Nutrition:

Energy (calories): 46 kcal

Protein: 0.64 g

Fat: 3.53 g

Carbohydrates: 3.3 g

Green Salad

Preparation time: 10 minutes

Cooking time: 10 minutes

Servings: 4

Ingredients:

- One tbsp. lemon juice
- Four red bell peppers
- One lettuce head, cut into strips
- Salt and black pepper to taste
- Three tbsp. coconut cream
- Two tbsp. olive oil
- 1 ounces rocket leaves

Direction:

Place bell pepper in your air fryer's basket.

Cook at the temperature of 400 degrees F for 10 minutes.

Transfer to a bowl and leave them aside to cool down.

Peel, cut them into strips and put them in a bowl.

Add rocket leaves and lettuce strips and toss.

In a bowl, mix oil with lemon juice, coconut cream, salt and pepper and whisk well.

Add over the salad, toss to coat divide between plates. Serve and enjoy!

Nutrition:

Energy (calories): 130 kcal

Protein: 2.71 g

Fat: 11.07 g

Carbohydrates: 7.54 g

Tomatoes Salad

Preparation time: 10 minutes
Cooking time: 20 minutes
Servings: 2

Ingredients:

- Two tomatoes halved
- Cooking spray
- Salt and black pepper to taste
- One tsp. parsley, chopped
- One tsp. basil, chopped
- One tsp. oregano, chopped
- One tsp. rosemary, chopped
- One cucumber, chopped
- One green onion, chopped

Direction:

Spray tomato halves with cooking oil.

Season with salt and pepper. Place them in your air fryer's basket.

Cook for 20 minutes at 320 degrees F.

Transfer tomatoes to a bowl.

Add parsley, basil, oregano, rosemary, cucumber and onion,

Toss, serve and enjoy!

Nutrition:

Energy (calories): 55 kcal

Protein: 2.59 g

Fat: 0.67 g

Carbohydrates: 11.62 g

Savoury French Mushroom Mix

Preparation time: 10 minutes

Cooking time: 25 minutes

Servings: 4

Ingredients:

- 2 pounds mushrooms, halved
- Two tsp. herbs de Provence
- ½ tsp. garlic powder
- One tbsp. olive oil

Direction:

Over a medium heat, heat a pan with the oil.

Add herbs and heat them for 2 minutes.

Add mushrooms and garlic powder and stir.

Introduce pan in your air fryer's basket and cook at 360 degrees F for 25 minutes.

Divide between plates. Serve and enjoy!

Nutrition:

Energy (calories): 81 kcal

Protein: 7.07 g

Fat: 4.15 g

Carbohydrates: 7.69 g

Zucchini and Squash Salad

Preparation time: 10 minutes

Cooking time: 25 minutes

Servings: 4

Ingredients:

- Six tsp. olive oil
- 1 pound zucchinis, cut into half-moons
- ½ pound carrots, cubed
- One yellow squash, cut into chunks
- Salt and white pepper to taste
- One tbsp. tarragon, chopped
- Two tbsp. tomato paste

Direction:

In your air fryer pan, mix oil with zucchinis, carrots, squash, salt, pepper, tarragon and tomato paste.

Cover and then cook at 400 degrees F for 25 minutes.

Divide between plates. Serve and enjoy!

Nutrition:

Energy (calories): 116 kcal

Protein: 4.18 g

Fat: 7.4 g
Carbohydrates: 10.99 g

Tasty Squash Stew

Preparation time: 10 minutes

Cooking time: 30 minutes

Servings: 8

Ingredients:

- Two carrots, chopped
- One yellow onion, chopped
- Two celery stalks, chopped
- Two green apples, cored, peeled and chopped
- Four garlic cloves, minced
- 2 cups butternut squash, peeled and cubed
- 6 ounces canned chickpeas, drained
- 6 ounces canned black beans, drained
- 7 ounces canned coconut milk
- Two tsp. chilli powder
- One tsp. oregano, dried
- One tbsp. cumin, ground
- 2 cups veggie stock
- Two tbsp. tomato paste
- Salt and black pepper to taste
- One tbsp. cilantro, chopped

Direction:

In your air fryer, mix carrots with onion, celery, apples, garlic, squash, chickpeas, black beans, coconut milk, chilli powder, oregano, cumin, stock, tomato paste, salt and pepper.

Stir, cover and cook at 370 degrees F for 30 minutes

Add cilantro and stir.

Divide into bowls and serve hot.

Nutrition:

Energy (calories): 112 kcal

Protein: 3.28 g

Fat: 2.37 g

Carbohydrates: 21.99 g

Chinese Green Beans Mix

Preparation time: 10 minutes

Cooking time: 30 minutes

Servings: 6

Ingredients:

- 1 pound green beans, halved
- 1 cup maple syrup
- 1 cup tomato sauce
- Four tbsp. stevia
- ¼ cup tomato paste
- ¼ cup mustard
- ¼ cup olive oil
- ¼ cup apple cider vinegar
- Two tbsp. coconut aminos

Direction:

In your air fryer, mix beans with maple syrup, tomato paste, stevia, tomato paste, mustard, oil, vinegar and amino.

Stir, cover and cook at 365 degrees F for 35 minutes.

Divide into bowls and serve hot.

Nutrition:

Energy (calories): 301 kcal

Protein: 2.92 g

Fat: 9.94 g

Carbohydrates: 51.5 g

Black Beans Mix

Preparation time: 10 minutes

Cooking time: 25 minutes

Servings: 6

Ingredients:

- One yellow onion, chopped
- One tbsp. olive oil
- One red bell pepper, chopped
- One jalapeno, chopped
- Two garlic cloves, minced
- One tsp. ginger, grated
- ½ tsp. cumin
- ½ tsp. allspice, ground
- ½ tsp. oregano, dried
- 30 ounces canned black beans, drained
- ½ tsp. stevia
- 1 cup of water
- A pinch of salt and black pepper
- 3 cups brown rice, cooked
- Two mangoes, peeled and chopped

Direction:

In your air fryer's pan, combine onion with the oil, bell pepper, jalapeno, garlic, ginger, cumin, allspice, oregano, black beans, stevia, water, salt and pepper.

Stir, cover and cook at 370 degrees F for 25 minutes.

Add rice and mangoes

Toss and divide between plates. Serve and enjoy!

Nutrition:

Energy (calories): 79 kcal

Protein: 2.14 g

Fat: 4.58 g

Carbohydrates: 9.28 g

Okra and Eggplant Stew

Preparation time: 10 minutes

Cooking time: 25 minutes

Servings: 10

Ingredients:

- 2 cups eggplant, cubed
- One butternut squash, peeled and cubed
- 2 cups zucchini, cubed
- 10 ounces tomato sauce
- One carrot, sliced
- One yellow onion, chopped
- ½ cup veggie stock
- 10 ounces okra
- 1/3 cup raisins
- Two garlic cloves, minced
- ½ tsp. turmeric powder
- ½ tsp. cumin, ground
- ½ tsp. red pepper flakes, crushed
- ¼ tsp. sweet paprika
- ¼ tsp. cinnamon powder

Direction:

In your air fryer, mix eggplant with squash, zucchini, tomato sauce, carrot, onion, okra, garlic, stock, raisins, turmeric, cumin, pepper flakes, paprika and cinnamon

Stir, cover and cook at 360 degrees for 5 minutes.

Divide into bowls. Serve and enjoy!

Nutrition:

Energy (calories): 39 kcal

Protein: 1.4 g

Fat: 1.17 g

Carbohydrates: 7 g

Savory White Beans Stew

Preparation time: 10 minutes

Cooking time: 20 minutes

Servings: 10

Ingredients:

- 2 pounds white beans, cooked
- Three celery stalks, chopped
- Two carrots, chopped
- One bay leaf
- One yellow onion, chopped
- Three garlic cloves, minced
- One tsp. rosemary, dried
- One tsp. oregano, dried
- One tsp. thyme, dried
- A drizzle of olive oil
- Salt and black pepper to the taste
- 28 ounces canned tomatoes, chopped
- 6 cups chard, chopped

Direction:

In your air fryer's pan, mix white beans with celery, carrots, bay leaf, onion, garlic, rosemary, oregano, thyme, oil, salt, pepper, tomatoes and chard.

Toss, cover and cook at 365 degrees F for 20 minutes.

Divide into bowls and serve.

Nutrition:

Energy (calories): 58 kcal

Protein: 2.43 g

Fat: 1.66 g

Carbohydrates: 10.31 g

Spinach and Lentils Mix

Preparation time: 10 minutes

Cooking time: 15 minutes

Servings: 8

Ingredients:

- 10 ounces spinach
- 2 cups canned lentils, drained
- One tbsp. garlic, minced
- 15 ounces canned tomatoes, chopped
- 2 cups cauliflower florets
- One tsp. ginger, grated
- One yellow onion, chopped
- Two tbsp. curry paste
- ½ tsp. cumin, ground
- ½ tsp. coriander, ground
- Two tsp. stevia
- A pinch of salt and black pepper
- ¼ cup cilantro, chopped
- One tbsp. lime juice

Direction

In a pan that suites your air fryer, mix spinach with lentils, garlic, tomatoes, cauliflower, ginger, onion, curry paste, cumin, coriander, stevia, salt, pepper and lime juice.

Stir, introduce in the air fryer and cook at 370 degrees F for 15 minutes.

Add cilantro and stir.

Divide into bowls. Serve and enjoy!

Nutrition:

Energy (calories): 68 kcal

Protein: 4.23 g

Fat: 1.9 g

Carbohydrates: 11.62 g

Cajun Mushrooms and Beans

Preparation time: 10 minutes

Cooking time: 15 minutes

Servings: 4

Ingredients:

- Two tbsp. olive oil
- One green bell pepper, chopped
- One yellow onion, chopped
- Two celery stalks, chopped
- Three garlic cloves, minced
- 15 ounces canned tomatoes, chopped
- 8 ounces white mushrooms, sliced
- 15 ounces canned kidney beans, drained
- One zucchini, chopped
- One tbsp. Cajun seasoning
- Salt and black pepper to the taste

Direction:

In your air fryer's pan, mix oil with bell pepper, onion, celery, garlic, tomatoes, mushrooms, beans, zucchini, Cajun seasoning, salt and pepper.

Stir, cover and cook on at 370 degrees F for 15 minutes.

Divide the veggie mix between plates. Serve and enjoy!

Nutrition:

Energy (calories): 192 kcal

Protein: 5.01 g

Fat: 13.12 g

Carbohydrates: 15.83 g

Corn and Cabbage Salad

Preparation time: 10 minutes

Cooking time: 15 minutes

Servings: 4

Ingredients:

- One small yellow onion, chopped
- One tbsp. olive oil
- Two garlic cloves, minced
- One and ½ cups mushrooms, sliced
- Three tsp. ginger, grated
- A pinch of salt and black pepper
- 2 cups corn
- 4 cups red cabbage, chopped
- One tbsp. Nutritional yeast
- Two tsp. tomato paste
- One tsp. coconut aminos
- One tsp. sriracha sauce

Directions:

In your air fryer's pan, mix the oil with onion, garlic, mushrooms, ginger, salt, pepper, corn, cabbage, yeast and tomato paste.

Stir, cover and cook at 365 degrees F for 15 minutes.

Add sriracha sauce and amino, stir, divide between plates. Serve and enjoy!

Nutrition:

Energy (calories): 387 kcal

Protein: 10.9 g

Fat: 7.57 g

Carbohydrates: 73.28 g

Wintergreen Beans

Preparation time: 10 minutes
Cooking time: 16 minutes
Servings: 4

Ingredients:
- One small yellow onion, chopped
- One tbsp. olive oil
- Two garlic cloves, minced
- One and ½ cups mushrooms, sliced
- Three tsp. ginger, grated
- A pinch of salt and black pepper
- 2 cups corn
- 4 cups red cabbage, chopped
- One tbsp. Nutritional yeast
- Two tsp. tomato paste
- One tsp. coconut aminos
- One tsp. sriracha sauce
- 1½ cups yellow onion, chopped
- 1 pound green beans, halved
- 4 ounces canned tomatoes, chopped
- Four garlic cloves, chopped
- Two tsp. oregano, dried

- One jalapeno, chopped
- Salt and black pepper to taste
- 1½ tsp. cumin, ground
- One tbsp. olive oil

Direction:

Preheat your air fryer at 365 degrees F temperature.

Add oil to the pan; also add onion, green beans, tomatoes, garlic, oregano, jalapeno, salt, pepper and cumin.

Cover and cook for 16 minutes.

Divide between plates. Serve and enjoy!

Nutrition:

Energy (calories): 503 kcal

Protein: 13.31 g

Fat: 15.3 g

Carbohydrates: 84.48 g

Green Beans Casserole

Preparation time: 10 minutes

Cooking time: 20 minutes

Servings: 4

Ingredients:

- One tsp. olive oil
- Two red chillies, dried
- ¼ tsp. fenugreek seeds
- ½ tsp. black mustard seeds
- Ten curry leaves, chopped
- ½ cup red onion, chopped
- Three garlic cloves, minced
- Two tsp. coriander powder
- Two tomatoes, chopped
- 2 cups eggplant, chopped
- ½ tsp. turmeric powder
- ½ cup green bell pepper, chopped
- A pinch of salt and black pepper
- 1 cup green beans, trimmed and halved
- Two tsp. tamarind paste
- One tbsp. cilantro, chopped

Direction:

Prepare baking dish that fits your air fryer combines the oil with chillies, fenugreek seeds, black mustard seeds, curry leaves, onion, coriander, tomatoes, eggplant, turmeric, green bell pepper, salt, pepper, green beans, tamarind paste and cilantro.

Toss and put in your air fryer.

Cook at 365 degrees F temperature for 20 minutes.

Divide between plates. Serve and enjoy!

Nutrition:

Energy (calories): 57 kcal

Fat: 1.7 g

Carbohydrates: 10.21 g

Vegan Fruits

Lemon Cream Bars

Preparation time: 25 minutes

Cooking time: 22 minutes

Servings: 6

Ingredients:

- 4 tablespoons coconut oil, melted
- ¼ teaspoon plus 1 pinch of kosher salt
- 1 teaspoon pure vanilla extract
- ½ cup plus 3 tablespoons granulated sugar
- ½ cup plus 2 tablespoons all-purpose flour
- ¼ cup freshly squeezed lemon juice
- Zest of 1 lemon
- ½ cup canned coconut cream
- 4 tablespoons cornstarch
- Powdered sugar, to taste

Directions:

Set the air fryer temp to 350°F (180°C).

In a prepared medium bowl, combine the coconut oil, ¼ teaspoon of salt, vanilla extract, and 3 tablespoons of sugar. Mix the flour until it forms a smooth dough. Transfer the mixture to a baking dish and gently press the dough to cover the bottom.

Place the dish in the fryer basket and bake until golden, about 10 minutes. Remove the crust from the fryer basket and set aside to cool slightly.

Using medium saucepan on the stovetop over medium heat, combine the lemon juice and zest, coconut cream, the pinch of kosher salt, and the remaining ½ cup of sugar,. Whisk in the cornstarch and cook until thickened, about 5 minutes. Pour the lemon mixture over the crust.

Place the dish in the fryer basket and cook until the mixture is bubbly and almost completely set, about 10 to 12 minutes.

Remove the dish from the fryer basket and set aside to cool completely. Transfer the dish to the refrigerator for at least 4 hours. Dust with the powdered sugar and then slice into 6 bars before serving.

Nutrition:

Energy (calories): 241 kcal

Protein: 1.88 g

Fat: 16.15 g

Carbohydrates: 23.8 g

Peanut Butter Cookies

Preparation time: 10 minutes

Cooking time: 10 minutes

Servings: 18 cookies

Ingredients:

- 1 tablespoon ground flaxseed
- 3 tablespoons water
- 1 cup creamy peanut butter
- ¾ cup light brown sugar
- 2/3 cup all-purpose flour
- 1 teaspoon baking soda
- ½ teaspoon kosher salt

Directions:

In a prepared small bowl, combine the flaxseed and water in a small bowl. Mix well and then set aside for 5 minutes.

Using another large bowl, combine the peanut butter and brown sugar. Add the flaxseed mixture, flour, baking soda, and salt. Mix until a soft dough forms. Refrigerate the dough, for at least 20 minutes.

Set the air fryer temp to 330°F (166°C). Spray the fryer basket using vegan nonstick cooking spray.

To roll the dough into 18 equally-sized balls, use a small scoop or tablespoon. Use a fork to press a diagonal hash mark into each ball.

Working in batches, place 9 balls in the fryer basket and cook until slightly golden, about 5 minutes.

Before it serves, move the cookies to a wire rack to cool.

Nutrition:

Energy (calories): 223 kcal

Protein: 5.83 g

Fat: 9.25 g

Carbohydrates: 28.78 g

Peach and Cherry Pies

Preparation time: 30 minutes

Cooking time: 20 minutes

Servings: 12 pies

Ingredients

- Dough:
- 2 cups self-rising flour
- ¼ cup all-vegetable shortening
- ¾ cup almond milk
- Filling:
- ¼ cup sugar
- 1 tablespoon cornstarch
- 3½ cups diced fresh peaches
- ½ cup dried cherries
- ½ cup sliced almonds
- 1 tablespoon lemon juice
- ¼–½ cup all-purpose white flour for work surface
- Oil for misting or cooking spray

Directions:

Pour the flour into a prepared large bowl and, using a pastry blender, cut the shortening into it.

Stir in the almond milk until a soft dough forms and set aside.

In a separate bowl, stir the filling Ingredients together and set aside.

Divide the dough into 12 equal-size portions and roll them into balls.

On a sheet of wax paper, sprinkle 1 tablespoon of flour.

On the wax paper with flour, roll one ball of dough out to a circle about 4½ to 5 inches in diameter. Use additional flour as needed to prevent the dough from sticking.

Place a heaping tablespoon of filling on the dough.

Using a pastry brush or using your finger dipped in water, moisten the inside edge of the dough all around.

Fold the dough to make a half-moon shape, press to seal it, and use a fork to crimp the edges shut.

Repeat steps 6 through 9 to make 3 more pies.

Mist both sides of the pies with oil or cooking spray and place in the air fryer basket.

Cook at 360°F (182°C) for 18 to 20 minutes, until the crust lightly browns.

Repeat steps 6–12 twice more to make the remaining pies.

Nutrition:

Energy (calories): 200 kcal

Protein: 2.86 g

Fat: 4.8 g

Carbohydrates: 37.79 g

Peach Yogurt Pudding Cake

Preparation time: 10 minutes

Cooking time: 35 minutes

Servings: 8

Ingredients:

- 1 (8-ounce / 227-g) can diced peaches packed in juice, drained
- Oil for misting or cooking spray
- ¼ cup silken tofu
- 2 tablespoons water
- 1 cup self-rising flour
- ¼ teaspoon baking soda
- ½ cup sugar
- 2 tablespoons oil
- 1 (5.3-ounce / 150 g) container vegan peach yogurt
- ¼ cup almond milk
- ¼ teaspoon almond extract

Directions:

Preheat the air fryer to 330°F (166°C).

Place the drained peaches in a single layer on several layers of paper towels, and cover with more paper towels to eliminate the excess moisture.

Spray the air fryer baking pan with oil or cooking spray.

In a prepared medium bowl, using a wire whisk, mix the silken tofu with the water.

Add the remaining Ingredients, including the peaches, and whisk until well mixed.

Pour the batter into the air fryer baking pan and cook for 35 minutes or if the toothpick is inserted into the center of the cake comes out clean.

Let the cake rest for 10 minutes before removing it from the baking pan.

Nutrition:

Energy (calories): 147 kcal

Protein: 2.25 g

Fat: 4.24 g

Carbohydrates: 25.2 g

Apple Crisp with Lemon

Preparation time: 10 minutes

Cooking time: 30 minutes

Servings: 4

Ingredients:

- The Topping:
- 2 tablespoons coconut oil
- ¼ cup plus 2 tablespoons of whole-wheat pastry flour (or gluten-free all-purpose flour)
- ¼ cup coconut sugar
- 1/8 teaspoon sea salt
- The Filling:
- 2 cups finely chopped (or thinly sliced) apples (no need to peel)
- 3 tablespoons water
- ½ tablespoon lemon juice
- ¾ teaspoon cinnamon

Directions:

To Make the Topping

In a bowl, combine the oil, flour, sugar, and salt. Mix the Ingredients together thoroughly, either with your hands or a spoon. The mixture should be crumbly; if it's not, place it in the fridge until it solidifies a bit.

To Make the Filling

In a 6-inch round, 2-inch deep baking pan, stir the apples with the water, lemon juice, and cinnamon until well combined.

Crumble the chilled topping over the apples. Bake or cook for about 30 minutes, or until the apples are tender and the crumble is crunchy and nicely browned. Serve immediately on its own or topped with nondairy milk, vegan ice cream, or nondairy whipped cream.

Nutrition:

Energy (calories): 139 kcal

Protein: 0.96 g

Fat: 6.97 g

Carbohydrates: 19.65 g

Plum Cake

Preparation time: 10 minutes

Cooking time: 30 minutes

Servings: 8

Ingredients:

- 4 plums pitted and chopped.
- 1 ½ cups almond flour
- ½ cup coconut flour
- ¾ cup almond milk
- ½ cup vegan butter, soft
- ¾ cup Silken Tofu
- ½ cup swerve
- 1 tbsp. vanilla extract
- 2 tsp. baking powder
- ¼ tsp. almond extract

Directions:

Prepare a bowl and mix all the Ingredients and whisk well.

Pour this into a cake pan that fits the air fryer after you've lined it with parchment paper, put the pan in the machine and cook at 370°F for 30 minutes.

Cool the cake down, slice and serve

Nutrition:

Calories: 183

Fat: 4g

Fiber: 3g

Carbs: 4g

Protein: 7g

Baked Plums

Preparation time: 5 minutes

Cooking time: 20 minutes

Servings: 6

Ingredients:

- 6 plums; cut into wedges
- 10 drops of stevia
- Zest of 1 lemon, grated
- 2 tbsp. water
- 1 tsp. ginger, ground
- ½ tsp. cinnamon powder

Directions:

In a pan that fits the air fryer, combine the plums with the rest of the Ingredients, toss gently.

Put the pan inside the air fryer and cook at 360°F for 20 minutes. Serve cold

Nutrition:

Calories: 170

Fat: 5g

Fiber: 1g

Carbs: 3g

Protein: 5g

Chocolate Strawberry Cups

Preparation time: 5 minutes
Cooking time: 10 minutes
Servings: 8

Ingredients:

- 16 strawberries; halved
- 2 cups chocolate chips; melted
- 2 tbsp. coconut oil

Directions:

In a pan which fits your air fryer, mix the strawberries with the oil and the melted chocolate chips, toss gently, put the pan in the air fryer and cook at 340°F for 10 minutes.

Divide into cups and serve cold

Nutrition:

Calories: 162

Fat: 5g

Fiber: 3g

Carbs: 5g

Protein: 6g

Fried Banana Slices

Preparation time: 15 minutes

Cooking time: 15 minutes

Servings: 8

Ingredients:

- 4 medium peeled ripe bananas, cut into 4 pieces lengthwise
- 1/3 cup rice flour, divided
- 4 tbsp. cornflour
- 2 tbsp. desiccated coconut
- ½ tsp. baking powder
- ½ tsp. vegan ground cardamom
- A pinch of salt

Directions:

Preheat the Air fryer to 390 0 F and grease an Air fryer basket.

Mix coconut, two tbsp. of rice flour, cornflour, baking powder, cardamom, and salt in a shallow bowl. Stir in the water gradually and then mix until a smooth mixture is formed.

Place the remaining rice flour in a second bowl and dip it in the coconut mixture.

Dredge in the rice flour and arrange the banana slices into the Air fryer basket in a single layer.

Cook for about 15 minutes, flipping once in between and dish out onto plates to serve.

Nutrition:

Calories: 260

Fat: 6g

Carbohydrates: 51.2g

Sugar: 17.6g

Protein: 4.6g

Sodium: 49mg

Vegan Dessert

Vanilla Cupcakes

Preparation time: 5 minutes

Cooking time: 15 minutes

Servings: 4

Ingredients:

- 2 cups wheat flour
- 1 ½ cup almond milk
- ½ tsp. baking powder
- ½ tsp. baking soda
- 2 tbsp. butter
- 1 tbsp. maple syrup
- 3 tbsp. vanilla extract
- 2 tsp. vinegar
- muffin cups

Directions:

Combine the Ingredients: except milk to create a crumbly blend. Add this milk to the mixture and make a batter and pour into the muffin cups. Preheat the fryer to 300 F and cook for 15 minutes.

Check whether they are done using a toothpick.

Nutrition:

Calories 161

Fat 5.6g

Protein 7.2g

Delectable Pear Muffins

Preparation time: 5 minutes

Cooking time: 15 minutes

Servings: 4

Ingredients:

- 2 cups All-purpose flour
- 1 ½ cup almond milk
- ½ tsp. baking powder
- ½ tsp. baking soda
- 2 tbsp. vegan butter
- 2 tbsp. sugar
- 2 cups sliced pears
- muffin cups

Directions:

Combine the Ingredients: except milk to create a crumbly blend. Add this milk to the mixture and make a batter and pour into the muffin cups. Preheat the fryer to 300 F and cook for 15 minutes.

Check whether they are done using a toothpick.

Nutrition:

Calories 114

Fat 4.8g

Protein 6.1g

Mini Rosemary Cornbread

Preparation time: 15 minutes
Cooking time: 25 minutes
Servings: 6

Ingredients:

- ¾ cup fine yellow cornmeal
- ½ cup sorghum flour
- ¼ cup tapioca starch
- ½ tsp. xanthan gum
- 2 tsp. baking powder
- ¼ cup granulated sugar
- ¼ tsp. salt
- 1 cup plain almond milk
- 3 tbsp. olive oil
- 2 tsp. fresh rosemary, minced

Directions:

In a prepared large bowl, mix the flour, cornmeal, starch, sugar, xanthan gum, baking powder, and salt.

Add the almond milk, oil, and rosemary. Mix until well combined.

Put the mixture into four greased ramekins evenly.

Press the "Power Button" of the Air Fry Oven and turn the dial to select the "Air Fry" mode.

Press the Time button and set the Cooking time to 25 minutes.

Now push the Temp button and rotate the dial to set the temperature at 400 degrees F.

Press the "Start/Pause" button to start.

When the unit beeps to show that it is preheated, open the lid.

Arrange the pan in "Air Fry Basket" and insert it in the oven.

Place the ramekins onto a wire rack for about 10-15 minutes.

Carefully invert the bread onto a wire rack to cool completely before serving.

Nutrition:

Calories 220

Total Fat 8.5 g

Carbs 35.5 g

Fiber 2.8 g

Sugar 8.6 g

Protein 2.8 g

Carrot Mug Cake

Preparation time: 15 minutes

Cooking time: 20 minutes

Serving: 1

Ingredients:

- ¼ cup whole-wheat pastry flour
- 1 tbsp. coconut sugar
- ¼ tsp. baking powder
- 1/8 tsp. ground cinnamon
- 1/8 tsp. ground ginger
- Pinch of ground cloves
- Pinch of ground allspice
- Pinch of salt
- 2 tbsp. plus two tsp. unsweetened almond milk
- 2 tbsp. carrot, peeled and grated
- 2 tbsp. walnuts, chopped
- 1 tbsp. raisins
- 2 tsp. applesauce

Directions:

In a prepared bowl, mix the flour, sugar, baking powder, spices and salt.

Add the remaining Ingredients and mix until well combined.

Place the mixture into a lightly greased ramekin.

Press the "Power Button" of Air Fry Oven and turn the dial to select the "Air Bake" mode.

Press the Time button and turn the dial to set the Cooking time to 20 minutes.

Now push the Temp button and rotate the dial to set the temperature at 350 degrees F.

Press the "Start/Pause" button to start.

When the unit beeps to show that it is preheated, open the lid.

Arrange the ramekin over the "Wire Rack" and insert in the oven.

Place the ramekin onto a wire rack to cool slightly before serving.

Nutrition:

Calories 301

Total Fat 10.1 g

Total Carbs 48.6 g

Fiber 3.2 g

Sugar 19.4 g

Protein 7.6 g

Simple Basil Tomatoes

Preparation time: 10 minutes

Cooking time: 10 minutes

Servings: 2

Ingredients:

- 3 tomatoes
- Olive oil cooking spray
- Salt and pepper to taste
- 1 tbsp. fresh basil, chopped

Directions:

Cut tomatoes in halves and drizzle them generously with cooking spray

Sprinkle salt, pepper, and basil

Press "Power Button" on your Air Fryer and select "Air Fry" mode

Press the Time Button and set time to 20 minutes

Push Temp Button and set temp to 320 degrees F

Press the "Start/Pause" button and start the device

Once the appliance beeps to indicated that it is pre-heated, arrange tomatoes in the Air Fryer cooking basket, let them cook

Once done, serve warm and enjoy!

Nutrition:

Calories: 34

Fat: 0.4 g

Saturated Fat: 0.1 g

Carbohydrates: 7 g

Fiber: 2 g

Sodium: 87 mg

Protein: 1.7 g

Cumin and Squash Chili

Preparation time: 10 minutes

Cooking time: 16 minutes

Servings: 4

Ingredients:

- 1 medium butternut squash
- 2 tsp. cumin seeds
- 1 large pinch chili flakes
- 1 tbsp. olive oil
- 1 and ½ ounces pine nuts
- 1 small bunch fresh coriander, chopped

Directions:

Take the squash and slice it

Remove seeds and cut into smaller chunks

Take a bowl and add chunked squash, spice and oil

Mix well

Pre-heat your Fryer to 360 degrees F and add the squash to the cooking basket in "AIR FRY" mode

Roast for 20 minutes, making sure to shake the basket from time to time to avoid burning

Take a pan and place it over medium heat, add pine nuts to the pan and dry toast for 2 minutes

Sprinkle nuts on top of the squash and serve

Enjoy!

Nutrition:

Calories: 339

Fat: 4 g

Saturated Fat: 1 g

Carbohydrates: 40 g

Fiber: 17 g

Sodium: 525 mg

Protein: 17 g

Dates Pudding

Preparation time: 5 minutes

Cooking time: 10 minutes

Servings:

Ingredients:

- 3 tbsp. Coconut sugar
- 2 tbsp. custard powder
- 3 tbsp. unsalted butter
- 1 cup pitted and sliced dates
- 1 tbsp. sugar

Directions:

Boil the milk and sugar in a pan and add the icing cream, followed by the dates and mix until you get a thick mixture. Add the sliced fruit to the mixture—Preheat the fryer to 300 degrees Fahrenheit for five minutes. Put the dish in the basket and reduce the temperature to 250 degrees Fahrenheit. Cook for ten minutes and let cool.

Nutrition:

Calories 122

Fat 4.6g

Protein 6.3g

Mini Lava Cakes

Preparation time: 10 minutes
Cooking time: 20 minutes
Servings: 3

Ingredients:

- ¼ cup Vegan Buttermilk
- Four tbsp. sugar
- Two tbsp. olive oil
- Four tbsp. almond milk
- Four tbsp. flour
- One tbsp. cocoa powder
- ½ tsp. baking powder
- ½ tsp. orange zest

Directions:

In a bowl, mix the flax egg with sugar, oil, milk, flour, salt, cocoa powder, baking powder and orange zest, stir very well and pour this into greased ramekins.

Add ramekins to your air fryer and cook at 320 degrees F for 20 minutes.

Serve lava cakes warm.

Enjoy!

Nutrition:

Calories 201

Fat 7

Fiber 8

Carbs 23

Protein 4

Vegan Snacks

Banana Chips

Preparation time: 10 minutes
Cooking time: 10 minutes
Servings: 4

Ingredients:

- Four bananas, peeled and sliced into thin pieces
- A drizzle of olive oil
- A pinch of black pepper

Directions:

Put banana slices in your air fryer, drizzle the oil, season with pepper, toss to coat gently and cook at 360 degrees for 10 minutes.

Serve as a snack. Enjoy!

Nutrition:

Calories 100

Fat 7g

Fiber 1g

Carbs 20g

Protein 1 g

Cabbage Rolls

Preparation time: 10 minutes

Cooking time: 25 minutes

Servings: 8

Ingredients:

- 2 cups cabbage, chopped
- Two yellow onions, chopped
- One carrot, chopped
- ½ red bell pepper, chopped
- 1-inch piece ginger, grated
- Eight garlic cloves, minced
- Salt and black pepper to the taste
- 1 tsp. coconut aminos
- 2 tbsp. olive oil
- Ten vegan spring roll sheets
- Cooking spray
- 2 tbsp. Cornflour mixed with 1 tbsp. water

Directions:

Heat a pan with the oil over medium-high heat, add cabbage, onions, carrots, bell pepper, ginger, garlic, salt, pepper and amino, stir, cook for 4 minutes take off the heat.

Cut each spring roll sheet and cut it into four pieces.

Place 1 tbsp. Veggie mix in one corner, roll and fold edges.

Repeat this with the rest of the rolls, place them in your air fryer's basket, grease them with cooking oil and cook at 360 degrees F for 10 minutes on each side.

Arrange on a plate and then serve as an appetizer.

Enjoy!

Nutrition:

Calories 150

Fat 3g

Fiber 4g

Carbs 7g

Protein 2g

Tortilla Chips

Preparation time: 10 minutes

Cooking time: 4 minutes

Servings: 4

Ingredients:

- Eight corn tortillas, each cut into triangles
- Salt and black pepper to the taste
- 1 tbsp. olive oil

Directions:

Brush tortilla chips with the oil, place them in your air fryer's basket and cook for 4 minutes at 400 degrees F

Serve them with salt and pepper sprinkled all over.

Enjoy!

Nutrition:

Calories 53g

Fat 1g

Fiber 1.5g

Carbs 10g

Protein 2 g

Chickpeas Snack

Preparation time: 10 minutes

Cooking time: 20 minutes

Servings: 4

Ingredients:

- 15 ounces canned chickpeas, drained
- ½ tsp. cumin, ground
- 1 tbsp. olive oil
- 1 tsp. smoked paprika
- Salt and black pepper to the taste

Directions:

In a bowl, mix chickpeas with oil, cumin, paprika, salt and pepper, toss to coat, place them in the fryer's basket, cook at 390 degrees F for 10 minutes, and transfer a bowl.

Serve as a snack

Enjoy!

Nutrition:

Calories 140

Fat 1g

Fiber 6g

Carbs 20g

Protein 6g

Vegan Bread and Pizza

Beer Bread (Vegan)

Preparation time: 10 minutes

Cooking time: 45 minutes

Servings: 4

Ingredients:

- 225 g wheat flour
- 150 ml dark beer (or malt beer)
- 75 g sourdough
- 10 g yeast
- 1 tbsp. salt
- For the rye sourdough:
- 75 g rye flour
- 75 ml water (lukewarm)

Direction:

For a successful beer bread, the sourdough must first be prepared! To do this, mix rye flour and lukewarm water into a dough and cover and leave to rest in a warm place for 12 hours.

As soon as the sourdough is left to rest, dissolve the yeast and salt in 3 tbsp. Of dark beer until bubbles form. Then add the sourdough, wheat flour and the remaining dark beer and knead for 8 minutes.

Cover again the dough and then let it rest in a warm place for 1-2 hours. Then either put the dough in the hot air fryer's baking pan without further processing or shape it like a loaf and place it on the grid insert. Bake bread for 5 minutes at 200 ° C, then reduce the baking temperature to 180 ° C and bake for another 25 minutes.

Now and then, brush the bread with a little water to have excellent, shiny crust forms.

Nutrition:

Energy (calories): 326 kcal

Protein: 10.46 g

Fat: 1.31 g

Carbohydrates: 67.31 g

Fitness Bread (Vegan)

Preparation time: 10 minutes

Cooking time: 80 minutes

Servings: 1 bread

Ingredients:

- 150 g whole wheat flour
- 150 g wholemeal rye flour
- 1 tbsp. agave syrup, alternatively also maple syrup
- 25 g yeast
- 1 tsp. salt
- 1 tbsp. flaxseed oil
- 40 g chopped walnuts
- 35 g chopped pumpkin seeds
- 50 g dried fruit of your choice cut into pieces (dates, raisins, etc.)
- Water for brushing

Directions:

Sieve wheat and rye flour and add salt. Dissolve the yeast in lukewarm water and mix in agave syrup. Add the flour and oil and knead everything into a soft dough. Then cover a clean kitchen towel with the dough and let it rest in a warm position for 30 minutes .

In the meantime, mix the chopped nuts and kernels with the dried fruit cut into pieces and, after the resting time, knead well into the dough.

Place the dough in the baking pan of the air fryer and cover it for another 15 minutes. Then program the air fryer to 200 ° C and bake the loaf for 5 minutes. Then reduce the temperature to 180 ° C and bake for another 55 minutes. Brush the bread with a little water now and then to create a friendly, shiny crust.

Nutrition:

Energy (calories): 927 kcal

Protein: 27.26 g

Fat: 31.24 g

Carbohydrates: 147.53 g

Wholegrain Bread (Vegan)

Preparation time: 10 minutes

Cooking time: 60 minutes

Servings: 1bread

Ingredients:

- 500 g whole wheat flour
- 150 g ready-made sourdough
- 100 g grain mixture
- 300 ml of lukewarm water
- One packet of dry yeast
- 2 tbsp. salt

Directions:

Put the flour, sourdough, salt, water, dry yeast and 2/3 of the grain mixture in a prepared large bowl and knead into a dough. Cover the dough in the bowl with a clean kitchen towel and leave in a warm place for an hour.

Line the air fryer with parchment paper and place the loaf on top. Brush the loaf surface with water and carefully press the rest of the grain mixture into the loaf.

Bake bread for 10 minutes at 200 ° C, and then reduce the temperature to 150 ° C and bake for another 40 minutes. Let the bread cool down well before eating.

Nutrition:

Energy (calories): 542 kcal

Protein: 17.27 g

Fat: 5.02 g

Carbohydrates: 114.68 g

Walnut Bread With Cranberries (Vegan)

Preparation time: 10 minutes

Cooking time: 40 minutes

Servings: 1bread

Ingredients:

- 500 g of wheat flour
- One yeast cube
- 250 ml of lukewarm water
- 1 tbsp. salt
- 100 g walnuts
- 100 g cranberries, dried

Directions:

In a prepared bowl, mix the flour and salt and create a well in the middle. Pour the yeast into the well and pour lukewarm water over it. Let rest for 10 minutes.

Then add walnuts and cranberries and knead everything into a dough. Grease the bread pan and dust with flour. Alternatively line with baking paper.

Now cover the bread pan with a clean kitchen towel and let rise in a warm place for 60 minutes.

Then bake for 30-35 minutes at 200 ° C.

Nutrition:

Energy (calories): 632 kcal

Protein: 16.72 g

Fat: 17.55 g

Carbohydrates: 102.2 g

Vegan Main Dishes

Cauliflower Rice

Preparation time: 10 minutes

Cooking time: 20 minutes

Servings: 3

Temperature: 370degreesF

Ingredients:

- For the tofu
- Two carrots, diced
- ½ cup onion, diced
- 2 tbsp. soy sauce
- 1 tsp. turmeric
- ½ block firm tofu, crumbled
- For the rice
- 3 cups riced cauliflower
- 2 tbsp. sodium soy sauce, reduced
- ½ cup broccoli, finely chopped
- 1 tbsp. rice vinegar
- ½ cup peas, frozen
- Two garlic cloves, minced

- One and ½ tsp. sesame oil, toasted
- 1 tbsp. ginger, minced
- ½ cup frozen peas
- 1 tbsp. rice vinegar

Directions:

Preheat and set the Air Fryer's temperature to 370 degrees F

Take a large bowl and add tofu alongside remaining tofu Ingredients

Stir well to combine

Set in the Air Fryer to cook for 10 minutes

Take another bowl and add the remaining Ingredients

Stir them well

Transfer into the Air Fryer and cook 10 minutes more

Serve and enjoy!

Nutrition:

Calories: 153

Fat: 4g

Carbohydrates: 18g

Protein: 10g

Sweet Potato Cauliflower Patties

"In the mood for some patties? Just make them from cauliflower! They will be both healthy and fried!"

Preparation time: 15 minutes

Cooking time: 20 minutes

Servings: 1

Temperature: 400degreesF

Ingredients:

- 2 cups cauliflower florets
- 2 tbsp. arrowroot powder
- 1 tsp. garlic, minced
- One large sweet potato, peeled and chopped
- ¼ cup flaxseed, grounded
- 1 cup cilantro, packed
- ¼ tsp. cumin
- 2 tbsp. Ranch seasoning mix
- ¼ cup sunflower seeds
- ½ tsp. chilli powde r
- 1 cup cilantro, packed
- One green onion, chopped

- Salt and pepper
- Any dipping sauce for serving

Directions:

Preheat your Air Fryer and set the temperature at 400 degrees F

Add sweet potato, cauliflower, onion, garlic, and sizzle into your food processor

Blend until smooth

Mould the mixture into patties and place onto a greased baking sheet

Place into your freezer for 10 minutes

Then transfer into your Air Fryer

Cook for 20 minutes and flip after 10 minutes

Serve and enjoy!

Nutrition:

Calories: 85

Fat: 2.9g

Carbohydrates: 6g

Protein: 2.7g

Breaded Mushrooms

"Take your normal mushrooms and turn them into this crispy treat for all ages! Your kids are going to love you for this!"

Preparation time: 15 minutes
Cooking time: 7 minutes
Servings: 2
Temperature: 360degreesF

Ingredients:

- ½ pound button mushrooms
- 1 cup almond meal
- 1 Flax-Egg
- 1 cup almond flour
- 3 ounces cashew cheese
- Salt and pepper

Directions:

Preheat and set the Air Fryer's temperature to 360 degrees F

Take a shallow bowl and toss almond meal with cheese into it

Whisk flax egg in one bowl and spread flour in another

Wash mushrooms, then pat dry

Coat every mushroom with flour

Dip each of them in the flax egg first, then in breadcrumb

Spray with cooking oil and place back in the Air Fryer

Air fry these mushrooms for 7 minutes in your Air Fryer

Toss the mushrooms after 3 minutes

Once cooked, serve warm

Enjoy!

Nutrition:

Calories: 140

Fat: 9.2g

Carbohoydrates: 6.9g

Protein: 9.3g

Vegan Staples

Twice Baked Stuffed Idaho Potatoes

Preparation time: 20 minutes

Cooking time: 65 minutes

Servings: 4

Ingredients:

- 1 cup spinach, chopped, OR kale
- 1-2 tsp. of olive oil, optional
- 1/2 tsp. salt
- 1/4 cup unsweetened non-dairy milk
- 1/4 cup unsweetened vegan yogurt
- 1/4 tsp. pepper
- 2 Idaho® Russet Baking Potatoes, large-sized
- 2 tbsp. of Nutritional yeast
- Optional toppings:
- 1/4 cup vegan yogurt, unsweetened
- Parsley, or chives, or your choice of fresh herb, chopped

- Smoked salt and pepper

Directions:

Rub all sides of the potatoes with oil.

Preheat the air fryer to 390F, unless your air fryer model does not require preheating. When the air fryer is hot, put the potatoes in the basket and set the timer for 30 minutes. When the timer beeps, flip the potatoes and set the timer for 30 minutes. Depending on potato size, you may have to add 10-20 minutes more of **Cooking time**. The potatoes are done when a fork can be easily pierced into them. When the potatoes are already cooked, let them cool enough until you can handle them.

In a lengthwise manner, slice the potato into halves. Scoop out the middle portion carefully from each potato half, leaving enough for a stable shell of white part and skin.

Mashup the scooped-out potato and mix with the **Nutrition**al yeast, non-dairy milk, vegan yogurt, pepper, and salt until the mixture is smooth. Stir the spinach into the mixture and combine.

Put the potato mixture in the potato shells.

Depending on the potato size, you can fit 2-4 potato halves in the air fryer basket. Cook in batches, if needed.

Set the air fryer's temperature to 350 degrees F and set the timer for 5 minutes.

Serve. Top with your choice of toppings, if desired.

Nutrition:

Energy (calories): 210 kcal

Protein: 7.84 g

Fat: 3.35 g

Carbohydrates: 37.79 g

Falafel Balls

Preparation time: 30 minutes

Cooking time: 12 minutes

Servings: 3

Ingredients:

- One can (15 ounces) chickpeas, drained and then rinsed, OR 2 cups cooked chickpeas
- 1 cup rolled oats
- One lemon, freshly squeezed juice onl y
- 1 tbsp. flax meal
- 1 tsp. garlic powder
- 1 tsp. ground cumin
- 1/2 cup diced sweet onion
- 1/2 cup minced carrots
- 1/2 cup roasted salted cashews
- 1/2 tsp. turmeric
- 2 tbsp. olive oil
- 2 tbsp. soy sauce

Directions:

Put the olive oil into a large-sized frying pan and heat over medium-high heat. When the oil is hot, add the carrots and onions, and sauté for about 7 minutes or until softened. Transfer to a large-sized bowl.

Put the oats and cashews into a food processor. Process until the mixture resembles a coarse meal. With the carrot mixture, apply the oat mixture to the dish. Put the chickpeas into the food processor. Add the lemon juice and soy sauce and the puree until the combination is semi-smooth – chunks are alright. You may need to stop and drag the sides a couple of times to get the Ingredients moving. Transfer the chickpea mixture into the bowl with the mix of oat and carrot.

Add the spices and the flaxseed to the bowl. Using a fork, mix all Ingredients until well combined, mashing any large pieces of chickpeas in the process.

With your clean hands, divide the mixture into 12 portions and form the pieces into balls. In a single layer, arrange the balls in the air fryer basket.

Set the temperature to 370F and the timer for 12 minutes – shake the basket after 8 minutes.

Serve as desired – stuffed into pitas together with tahini dressing or serve with your preferred accompaniments.

Nutrition:

Energy (calories): 604 kcal

Protein: 18.44 g

Fat: 38.25 g

Carbohydrates: 64.59 g

Black Bean-Tomato Soup with Poblano Chili Rings

Preparation time: 20 minutes

Cooking time: 25 minutes

Servings: 6

Ingredients:

- For the soup:
- 4 cups black beans, cooked and puréed
- 3 Roma tomatoes, coarsely chopped
- Three cloves garlic
- 2 1/2 cups vegetable broth
- 1/2 white onion, medium-sized, coarsely chopped
- 1 to 2 tbsp. corn oil
- 1 tsp. salt
- One ancho chilli stemmed and then seeded
- 1 1/2 cups water
- For the poblano chilli rings:
- One poblano chilli, cut into 1/2-inch thick rings
- 1/2 cup garbanzo or white bean aquafaba
- 1/2 cup panko breadcrumbs, divided
- 1/2 tsp. salt, divided
- For garnishing:

- Poblano Chile Rings
- Ripe Hass avocado, chopped
- Tortilla strips or chips
- Vegan sour cream, vigorously whipped

Directions:

For the poblano chilli rings:

Toss 1/4 cup panko breadcrumbs with 1/4 tsp. Salt in a shallow bowl. Do the same with the remaining panko breadcrumbs and salt in another shallow bowl. Set aside one of the bowls with the panko breadcrumb mixture.

Dredge the chilli slices in the aquafaba and then coat with the breadcrumb mixture. The panko mixture will initially stick to the rings well, but after the first half of the calls, it will begin to clump and no longer stick well. When this happens, use the second bowl of panko mixture.

In a single layer, arrange the coated chilli slices in the air fryer basket – do not overlap. You may need to cook in batches.

Set the air fryer's temperature to 390 degrees F and the timer for 8 to 10 minutes – shake the basket after 5 minutes – you want the chillies soft, and the panko browned. Cook the next batches for about 6 to 8 minutes since the air fryer is already hot. Serve right away topped with your soup.

For the soup:

Put the ancho chilli, tomatoes, and water into a 3-quart pot and stir to combine. Turn the heat to medium heat and let simmer for about 10 minutes.

After 10 minutes, carefully transfer the soup to a blender. Add the onion and garlic into the blender and puree until smooth – hold down the blender's cover with a clean kitchen towel to prevent the top from exploding. If you want to achieve a completely smooth puree, press the puree through a strainer.

Wipe the pot clean. Put the oil into the pot and heat on medium-high flame or heat. Return the puree to the pot and cook for around 5 minutes, stirring slowly. After 5 minutes, turn the heat to medium. Add the pureed bean, salt, and broth. Simmer for 10 minutes, adding liquid if needed to make the soup creamy but not too thick. Serve garnished with poblano chilli rings and your preferred other garnishes.

Nutrition:
Energy (calories): 1046 kcal
Protein: 12.98 g
Fat: 98.89 g
Carbohydrates: 37.43 g

Seaweed Salad with Crispy Tofu and Veggies

Preparation time: 35 minutes

Cooking time: 18 minutes

Servings: 4

Ingredients:

- One batch of crispy tofu (starch the tofu once the wakame is on the stove)
- One cucumber, large-sized
- 1 Haas avocado, chopped
- 1/4 cup green onion, chopped
- 1/4 cup sesame seeds
- 1/4 cup shiitake sesame vinaigrette (I used Annie's Naturals)
- Two carrots, peeled
- Three strips of dried wakame

Directions:

Soak the wakame in water for 5 minutes. After soaking, drain and then chop the strips into the bite-sized piece. Boil a pot of water. When the water is boiling, put the wakame pieces and cook for 5 minutes. After cooking, drain the wakame pieces and put them in the refrigerator to chill.

Spiralize the carrots and cucumber. If you do not have sriracha, then just chop them.

Toss the cucumber and carrots with the chilled wakame. Top with tofu, avocado, green onion, and sesame seeds. Serve right away

Nutrition:

Energy (calories): 221 kcal

Protein: 5.58 g

Fat: 19.05 g

Carbohydrates: 11.18 g

Easy Keto Tomato Basil Soup

A creamy and delicious low carb tomato soup recipe that takes just minutes to prepare! Keto, Atkins, and gluten free – this is an easy and tasty soup that you can feel great about serving to your family!

Prep Time: 2 minutes Cook Time: 10 minutes Total Time: 12 minutes Servings: 6 servings

Ingredients

- 1 can (28 ounces) whole plum tomatoes (San Marzano preferred)
- 2 cups filtered water
- 1.5 teaspoons coarse kosher salt
- 1/2 teaspoon onion powder
- 1/4 teaspoon garlic powder
- 1 tablespoon butter
- 8 ounces mascarpone cheese
- 2 tablespoons granulated erythritol sweetener
- 1 teaspoon apple cider vinegar
- 1/4 teaspoon dried basil leaves

- 1/4 cup prepared basil pesto, plus more for garnish if desired

-

Instructions

Combine the canned tomatoes, water, salt, onion powder and garlic powder in a medium saucepan.

Bring to a boil over medium-high heat and then simmer for 2 minutes.

Remove from the heat and puree with an immersion blender until smooth (or transfer to a traditional blender and blend, then return blended soup to the pan.)

Return to the stove and add the butter and mascarpone cheese to the soup.

Stir over low heat until melted and creamy – about 2 minutes. Remove from the heat and stir in the sweetener, apple cider vinegar, dried basil, and pesto.

Serve warm.

Store any leftovers in a covered container in the refrigerator for up to 5 days, or in the freezer for up to three months.

Nutrition Info

Serving Size: 1 cup Calories: 258

Fat: 23g Carbohydrates: 6g Fiber: 3g

Protein: 4g

Asian Noodle Salad with Peanut Sauce

This easy vegetarian Keto Asian Noodle Salad can be made in advance for picnics, parties, or as meal prep for keto lunches all week! Low carb, Atkins, Paleo, gluten free, and can easily be made vegan

Prep Time: 10 minutes Total Time: 10 minutes Servings: 4 servings

Ingredients

For the salad:

- 1 cup shredded red cabbage
- 1 cup shredded green cabbage 1/4 cup chopped scallions
- 1/4 cup chopped cilantro
- 4 cups shiritake noodles (drained and rinsed) 1/4 cup chopped peanuts
- For the dressing:
- 2 tablespoons minced ginger 1 teaspoon minced garlic
- ½ cup filtered water
- 1 tablespoon lime juice

- 1 tablespoon toasted sesame oil
- 1 tablespoon wheat-free soy sauce
- 1 tablespoon fish sauce (or coconut aminos for vegan)
- ¼ cup sugar free peanut butter
- ¼ teaspoon cayenne pepper
- ½ teaspoon kosher salt
- 1 tablespoon granulated erythritol sweetener

Instructions

Combine all of the salad ingredients in a large bowl.

Combine all of the dressing ingredients in a blender or magic bullet.

Blend until smooth. Pour the dressing over the salad and toss to coat.

Serve immediately, or store in an airtight container in the refrigerator for up to 5 days. Do not freeze.

Nutrition Info

Serving Size: 1.5 cups Calories: 212

Fat: 16g Carbohydrates

www.ingramcontent.com/pod-product-compliance
Lightning Source LLC
Chambersburg PA
CBHW062119040426
42336CB00041B/2003